YOU CAN'T MAKE THIS STUFF UP!

TALES OF AN OBGYN

DR. LAURA A. KATZ

WAKEFIRE
PRESS

You Can't Make This Stuff Up!

Tales of an OBGYN

Copyright © 2022 by Dr. Laura A. Katz, MD

Cover Design by Dee Dee Book Covers

Author Photos by Michael LaHote (Award-winning photographer and fellow cancer survivor)

ISBNs:

978-1-950476-39-8 (paperback)

978-1-950476-40-4 (eBook)

❀ Created with Vellum

PROLOGUE

Hello everyone! My name is Dr. Laura A. Katz. This is my second venture in the author realm. I really got the bug after publishing my book *OK, It's My Turn Now* last year when I was fighting my battle with lymphoma.

Let me tell you a little bit about myself. I have been a solo practicing Obstetrician-Gynecologist, or OBGYN, for over 20 years. During that time, I have cared for women of all ages seven days a week, 24 hours a day. That's the reality when you are in practice by yourself. It sounds like a lot, but I have loved every minute of it. I have no regrets or complaints about my choice; I knew what I was signing up for.

As I have progressed in my career, I have noticed that patients and outsiders really don't seem to understand what the life of an OBGYN is all about. I think that leads to misconceptions, misunderstandings, and a general lack of empathy by the public for OBGYNs and, to be honest, all practicing physicians right now.

I hope that by sharing some insights into my world, you will see a new perspective and learn what it really takes to be a physician caring for patients today. Some of these stories are funny and some are very serious. They all share one thing in common: they are all valued lessons that have built the foundation for who I am as a person, and who I am as a physician. I am grateful to have experienced every one of them. This book comes straight from the heart. I hope you enjoy it. You truly *can't* make this stuff up.

PART I

THE BACK STORY

1

A CIRCUITOUS PATH

So, how does one become an OBGYN you ask? I mean, it's not like you wake up one day and realize that it is your dream to stare at vaginas all day long. It just doesn't happen that way. At least it didn't for me. My path was, at best, circuitous, but I ended up where I belonged eventually.

I will let you in on a little secret: I am really a musician at heart. My whole life had been spent with the intent to be a symphony violinist. Hours upon hours of practice, lots of lessons, winning national music competitions, studying all over the United States...all propelling me toward the goal of becoming a member of a professional symphony orchestra.

I even got as far as auditioning for music school, which were some of the most exciting moments of my life. I was sure that was what I wanted to do... and then I was not so sure. My mind started to race with all kinds of ridiculously practical thoughts. My dreams of being a symphony musician were interrupted by thoughts like, "Hey, there aren't many symphony jobs out there," and "These are lifetime positions, and nothing opens up until somebody moves or dies," and "How often does THAT happen?"

It's not that I was trying to chicken out of my dream before it started - I suddenly had a reality check on the practicality of it and the possibility of making a sustainable living. Further, I created a self-fulfilled prophecy - I thought about it to the point that I subconsciously threw an audition or two to eliminate those choices. I thought it would make my choice easier. Actually, it made it harder.

Nonetheless, I ended up deciding that I would go to a regular undergraduate school, get a regular degree, get an excellent job, and then I'd be able to afford to get a great instrument to play in the future. So, you see, music never really left my mind.

Fortunately, I had not relied on my musical talent alone in high school. I had good grades and test scores and was able to get into the undergraduate school of my choice. I decided to go to the University of Michigan. At the time, they had the best political science department in the country, so I thought I would major in that and then maybe go to law school.

Wrong! So wrong! I couldn't stand my political science classes. I didn't realize there could be a subject on this earth I was less interested in. (This is still true today. Political conversations tend to make me run in the opposite direction rather than participate.) I also realized that I had *no* interest in arguing in a courtroom all day.

However, I *was* interested in playing my violin as much as possible, even if it was no longer where I planned to take my career. So, I joined the campus orchestra as a non-music major. Ironically, I was heavily recruited to transfer to the music program, an offer I politely declined, but I kept playing. It was tempting though.

I started taking more science classes and soon, I was changing my major to biology, which was much more "me". However, I'd lost time and money spent on political science classes that didn't count towards my degree. I didn't realize at the time how hard it was going to be to finish all my college requirements in four years. They make it sound easy to just extend college to five or six years, but they don't tell you how much more it will cost! I ended up taking additional spring and summer semester classes just to make up enough credits without completely killing myself during the regular school year.

I followed my science interests all the way to taking the MCAT, which is the medical school admission test, and applying to medical school. At this point, I had decided that medical school was the right choice for me. I knew that I wanted to pursue medical school. That much I was sure of. I still didn't know which area of medicine that I wanted to study or practice. I thought I was going to be an allergist, because my own allergist had saved my life on several occasions. My path directing me away from allergy to OBGYN is a whole other story.

2

FINDING MY TRUE PATH

Wayne State! Great School! This was the catchphrase coined by the beloved alum Casey Kasem in a 1980s billboard - always one of my favorites. Well, Casey was right! Fortunately, the MCAT went well, and I got into Wayne State University in Detroit. It was my school of choice, and I was invited for early admission, so I accepted right away and tossed aside all my other upcoming interviews. I was sure this was the place for me.

Medical school was an experience I was not prepared for. I thought I had it tough in undergraduate with all the tests and studying and memorizing. Well, all the tests and studying and memorizing of college about fit into the first day of medical school. *Sheesh!*

I really had no idea that the first two years of med school would be a barrage of fast-paced, volume heavy, memorization of endless information. Further, most of that information I did not use later in practice or had to relearn as science evolves over time. There were so many fast-paced lectures that sometimes we had to subscribe to a note-taking service to ensure you truly had all the material we'd missed simply by not writing quickly enough. *Paying for notes?!*

I slogged my way through the first two years, biding my time to get to the clinical rotations. These are the rotations through various areas of medicine to help you decide what to do with the rest of your life. Surgery, internal medicine, OBGYN, and pediatrics are just a few of the options.

At the start of my clinical rotations, I was still pretty set on going into internal medicine, until I had my internal medicine rotation. No. No. It was not for me. The endless pondering and postulating were not a good fit. I realized that internist could spend hours espousing on just one aspect of a patient's health history, without ever reaching a conclusion or changing anything! I discovered quickly that action and variety were more my style. I am, however, grateful for the folks who *can* do it - I salute you.

I loved my Emergency Room rotation.! I was on fire during that one! I was in on trauma calls, throwing intravenous fluid drips (IVs) into drunk guys going through delirium tremens (DTs), and doing facial plastic flaps on people who had been hit with hockey pucks at a Red Wings game. It was an awesome, adrenaline-filled adventure. But there was no long-lasting patient connection; it was all shift work.

I had some incredible experiences, though. I'm convinced some of these incidents were TV-show worthy. For example, one night this guy came in short of breath and wheezing. He had a pneumothorax (a dropped or deflated lung). There were no other medical issues: his drug test was negative and there was not a scratch on him. The only thing I noticed was that he had a Band-Aid on his chest.

I, the pesky medical student, just couldn't let it go. I kept asking if we should take the Band-Aid off to see what was underneath. The attending physicians (who had completed their residency and practiced full-time at the hospital) kept brushing me off, telling me to be quiet. Finally, I couldn't take it anymore and I just reached over and ripped off the Band-Aid.

Just as they all started yelling at me, they noticed the huge stab wound underneath! There was the reason for his pneumothorax! I just stood there grinning as the rest of the attending physicians got to work and he was rushed to surgery. As it turned out, his girlfriend had stabbed him for cheating on her, then freaked out and called 911 because she felt guilty. How crazy is that?!

Still, with all that movie-worthy action, I still wanted something that was more than shift work. The ER was not for me either. Finally, I started my OBGYN rotation. *Oh, sweet ambrosia!* I had no idea the vast variety of experiences encompassed by this profession. To be an OBGYN was to perform surgery, medicine, obstetrics, oncology, and all things women's health in one specialty! The only time males were involved was for circumcisions. I was amazed!

The real clincher was my first delivery of a real live human baby. I was so filled with wonder that I cried on the spot, much to the amusement of the mother and the entire Obstetrics (OB) team. I didn't care. I just let the happy tears flow. I had found my calling.

3

HOW I MET MY HUSBAND

Wayne State had one more life-changing surprise waiting for me...my future husband! The last place I was looking for love was in medical school, but that's where I found it.

Actually, when I started medical school, I was fresh off of a "near engagement" with a long-term boyfriend. I cared deeply about him, but I didn't think our future was meant to be together. I knew I was going to be overwhelmed with work with medical school and we were going to be long-distance, in separate states. It just seemed impossible. I did not want to be the girl that had to say no to a proposal. I broke it off poorly and part of me still regrets the how, but not the why. I needed to start fresh and concentrate on school.

Well, the universe had other plans! I was concentrating on classes, but slowly, my future husband came into my focus. At first, he was just the guy that laughed a little too long at every joke. I mean a quality 30 seconds after everyone else was done. It was enough to make you cringe *and* marvel at his unbridled exuberance. He was also the guy who dressed up for class every day in the most fabulous 70s leisure suits you have ever seen. Oh, yes. He was "all that."

We didn't have much to talk about until we did: one day, I was in the cafeteria with my friends, and he walked over and just sat down. I said an awkward, "Hello," and he started talking to me. My friends and I were going to a Detroit Symphony concert in a few days and could not find anyone to use the last ticket – not everyone was interested.

Well, lo and behold, he *was*! He invited himself along with us so ticket wouldn't go unused. We thought, "Why not?" We knew he lived in a dangerous part of town, so we weren't interested in driving there. He met us at Orchestra Hall, showing up in this Pontiac Sunbird SE with a broken hatchback. He told me that "SE" stood for "sexy edition." I laughed and brushed it off.

We all went inside and enjoyed the concert. I had been a symphony geek for as long as I could remember, and I had a lot of stored useless knowledge about the orchestra. I didn't share it as a rule, because people in general were not interested, but he was! He was genuinely glued to every word.! I was surprised, but *still* didn't catch on yet that he was interested in me.

After the concert, we wanted to go dancing, but we wanted to get the heck out of Detroit and up to Royal Oak. He wanted to go too, so we asked him to drive his own car all the way up to Royal Oak to meet us. As it turns out, he liked to dance too! For all you ladies out there, you know it is a rarity to find a man who likes to dance so grab on when you find one.

We danced for hours, and he offered to take me home. My friend didn't mind and drove herself home. I got into the "sexy edition" Sunbird, and he announced that he would like to kiss me. *Oh!* Now I get it, he likes me! I thought, "What the heck!" and I let him kiss me.

He barely brushed my lower lip and I swear I floated for three days! That had never happened to me. Usually, I am the girl that "grows to love" someone over time. I never had an instant reaction like that before. On top of that, he took me home and we literally talked until dawn. Just like a movie! I have never fallen so hard and so fast for anyone... and I'm still incredibly in love with him today, 27 years later.

4

RESIDENCY IS SUPPOSED TO BE TOUGH!

Don't let anyone fool you, residency was a grueling affair back in the 90s. We endured unlimited working hours, no guaranteed education lectures, unlimited mandatory "on call" shifts, days off after being on call were prohibited, and unlimited patients you could be responsible for.

Today's residents have a limit to the number of hours they can work. They get predetermined and promised days off. They have a limit on the number of calls that they can take. They have set lecture days when they cannot be accessed at all for patient care. While I understand (and appreciate) the evolution of these programs to protect the physical and mental health of the students, I am concerned that we have gone too far past reality on the spectrum.

From the abundance of residents, I have worked with over the years, I have the impression that too many of them are not prepared for a realistic future in medicine. They seem to view it as a regular job, ideally nine to five, with a set, guaranteed salary, limited responsibility, and plenty of opportunity to be rested and refreshed for whatever they might have to do. They just don't seem to be as tough as they used to be, or as committed, in some cases.

In my reality, being a doctor is not just a job. It is a lifetime commitment. It is a responsibility for other human beings. It is not realistic to think you will always be rested before every surgery, every delivery or every possible task.

The reality is that patients don't know that you need a day off after you were on call. It doesn't matter. Emergencies will come up when they come up. They don't care about your schedule. I also get concerned about how limited specialties are becoming. Even OBGYN is on the chopping block for being split up into two residencies – Obstetrics and Gynecology.

I, for one, am glad that I experienced the full breadth of training for OBGYN. It would not have made sense to me to divide it, and I can't imagine picking between the two when I was in med school.

I guess the advice I would give to future OBGYN residents is to make sure you are going into this specialty for the right reasons. To me, the right reasons are because you love it, you are ready to work hard, you want to help women lead healthier better lives and have better pregnancies, and you are fully committed to making that happen.

It's not about the salary or worrying about your schedule. You can't allow yourself to resent your patients for robbing your free time. Do something else if that is the case. You are going to be exhausted sometimes, and *still* must handle that emergency. You need to know what you are signing up for.

I stress the importance of loving your job part more than ever because future generations of physicians face ever-decreasing reimbursements for services. Right now, reimbursement is about 30 percent, and comes about three months after you complete the service. Let me tell you, that is already hard to live on. It's only going to get harder from here. But I still love it.

I was fortunate to attend OBGYN residency at the Medical College of Ohio, now known as the University of Toledo. I applied for it based on the outstanding faculty, the balanced variety of rotations, and the ability to work in several hospitals where I could get plenty of surgical experience. I was fortunate enough to go through residency at a time when OBGYNs were briefly reclassified as primary care.

This meant my residency included training in family practice, surgical ICU, ER, and internal medicine, maternal fetal medicine and gynecologic oncology, in addition to my OBGYN training. It was fantastic. All of the extra knowledge and experience I gained has served me well all these years.

It was rough, but worth it. I felt ready for anything when I was done. I felt prepared for the real world. I am one of the few OBGYNs or surgeons that I know who does not have my stethoscope in the corner collecting dust. I examine a patient's whole body at every checkup, much to their surprise and their benefit.

5

TAKE AWAY LESSONS

Residency taught me a lot of things. It taught me about hard work. It taught me about responsibility. It taught me to never stop searching for the answer to seemingly impossible questions. It also taught me that you could never gain too much specific information about a patient... and those patients don't always tell you the truth or sometimes have their own agenda. It is up to you to get to the bottom of the issue for their own safety. I learned a lot about how to take a thorough and accurate patient history.

For example, one of the common questions we ask is regarding alcohol use (how often, how much, etc.). I have had patients tell me that they only have one drink a day, only to discover with more questioning that they meant an *entire* fifth of Jack Daniels a day. However, because I only asked how many drinks a day, they told me one - because they drink it all at one sitting. *See?* I could have missed out on key information if I hadn't asked more questions and I would have missed the opportunity to counsel her on the dangers of alcoholism.

Here's an example of a patient that really had an agenda we knew nothing about. We had to perform a cesarean section on a patient in her 20s for arrest of dilation. This means that her cervix would not dilate past a certain point. After the c section, her incision just would not heal and the bacteria we cultured were more consistent with bowel bacteria. Every time we would get it treated and healing, it would get infected again.

Finally, one day during rounds, we caught her picking her nose, wiping her butt, and then wiping it in her incision! This explained everything! She was contaminating her own incision! When we questioned her, it turned out that she was purposely infecting her own incision to delay her discharge because she did not want to go home.

We had no idea that she had social issues at home. We hadn't asked. We were able to get social services involved to help resolve some of the issues and educate the patient on the dangers of contaminating her incision and finally were able to get her home safely.

6

THE NIGHTLY RECAP

Talking in your sleep, or somniloquy, is a common type of parasomnia or abnormal behavior during sleep. Believe it or not, two out of three people talk in their sleep at some point in their lives. For most people, an episode lasts about 30 seconds. I must admit, I am in that group.

According to my husband, I am quite the avid sleep talker and residency provided endless things to discuss. Always the overachiever, I never limited my "episodes" to a mere 30 seconds. Apparently, I have talked him through crash c sections from start to finish, and my general opinions on how my day went and everyone I encountered, all without opening my eyes or even being fully conscious!

He tells me he just lays there and takes it all in, quiet as a church mouse, trying not to disturb me. As incredulous as it may seem, I am even funnier in my sleep - according to him - so eventually he loses control and starts laughing. At some point, he laughs so hard the bed starts shaking and it wakes me up. I am always completely startled and unaware of where I am for a minute, until I see him laughing his little keister off at me.

Every time, he shares all the crazy things I was saying. For years I thought he was just making it up, honest to God. Then I realized that there was no way he could possess the intimate level of detail unless he heard it from me. Finally, he recorded me and played it back the next morning. *Ok*, I was finally convinced.

THERE IS NOTHING YOU CAN SAY THAT'S GONNA SHOCK ME, BUT I KNOW YOU'RE GONNA TRY

You know the phrase, "I've heard it all."? Well, in 25 years of practicing OBGYN, this phrase has taken on a whole new meaning. Never in my life would I have imagined the situations I have been in or the things I have heard. Let me run down a few scenarios for you.

I have been propositioned during a pelvic exam, truly. The patient sat up in the middle of a pap smear and announced they wanted to have sex with me... right now! My response was a rather glib, "Well, that's a nice offer, but let's hold that thought for now until I finish your check up." Disappointed, the patient said they were only joking. *Um... who does that?*

I have had geriatric patients brag to me that they have the perfect solution to vaginal dryness: anal intercourse! Then, they look at me for a reaction. I can't bring myself to give them the satisfaction. I just look at them, smile and say, "Congratulations on your back up plan. That is really thinking outside the box." Then I move on. Sorry ladies, I will not be fazed!

I have had patients describe more than I *ever* wanted to know about their sexual practices in intimate (or gory) detail, describing everything from their fetishes to their 50 Shades of

Grey activities. I have to admit, I didn't realize some of them had it in them. Suddenly, they will stop mid-story and ask me "Oh, am I oversharing?" I say," No, honey. If you can't tell your gynecologist about this, who can you tell? I talk about vaginas all day."

The bottom line is *bring it on, people!* You can't really shock me - many before you have tried.

PART II

EARLY CAREER: GROUP PRACTICE

HOW IT STARTED (AND HOW IT ENDED)

Pursuing group practice was advocated for early in residency. We were advised about the easier lifestyle and balance it offers: there is less call, responsibilities are shared, expenses are shared, and usually your salary is contracted and set. But these are just a few of the potential perks.

The counter point to that is when you are on call, you are much busier because you are taking care of the patients of the whole group instead of just your patients. The shared responsibilities *sound* nice, but that means that your colleagues are also caring for your patients and there is a possibility that they won't provide the same level of care and attention you prefer.

Shared expenses also sound great, until you realize you will all have to pay the same amount into the pot every month, even if one of your partners uses three times the resources you do. Also, our purely academic residency professors failed to mention the chances of finding your perfect group of like-minded individuals with the same work philosophy and ethics is far less likely than you might think. It's also unrealistic to go into a group practice thinking that you can change everyone for the better.

You can't. I tried.

I made all the mistakes I didn't know were mistakes at the time. I jumped right into a group practice that I respected, knowing there were changes that needed to be made. I thought I could make those changes happen all by myself. I respected all those physicians. They would listen to me, right? Nope.

I joined a well-established group practice of physicians who were very set in their ways. I grew close with all of them, and I learned a ton. At first, things were great. We all got along. It was fun having partners to operate with. I didn't even mind the really busy on-call days because they were so much farther apart than I was used to. I really benefitted from all of their wisdom.

Then, slowly, everything began to change. As I got busier, I got the impression some of my partners became jealous of me. There were arguments over which patients would be assigned to my schedule. It was a problem if some patients decided they wanted to see me instead. Please understand, I have never in my life solicited a patient from another provider. It is just not my style. It still isn't. Still, the misconception grew, and it became a problem, despite my input. I just dealt with it and kept going.

Then, another issue reared its ugly head. One of my partners, whom I was closest to, started developing some health issues that were going to severely impair their ability to practice medicine. I took it upon myself to try to privately help them, an effort which was angrily rebuffed. In good conscience, I could not let this issue go.

I brought it to the group and got nowhere. No one wanted to be involved. I got the impression that certain members of the group were more concerned about losing a body in the call schedule than helping a colleague before something awful happened. I was worried that both my colleague and patients were going to get hurt. It just didn't have to be that way.

After that, everything started to fall apart. I felt like I was treated differently: my work relationships suffered, and my patient schedule mysteriously decreased. I knew that it was time for me to go before things got any worse. I was crushed. I did not want to leave, but I knew it was the right thing to do.

It was not going to be easy. I had to sign what's called a restriction of covenant, which meant that I would not be able to work anywhere else within a certain mile radius for at least a year. This also meant that I couldn't work in my hometown for the time being. It was a year and a half before I was able to start working again.

9

HELP, I'M TRAPPED!

One long, tiring OBGYN day, I was seeing a ton of patients in my group practice. In an employed group practice, there is less control over how many patients there are to see in a day. It is ingrained in your head that in order to keep up with the productivity scale, more is more. We were expected to accept our schedule, keep our heads down, and get those people seen no matter what. Needless to say, this is a concept I was happy to toss out the window when I switched to private practice.

So, there I was, seeing too many patients in too little time. The end of the day finally approached, and a genuinely nice lady was my last patient of the day. She had been put in one of my regular-sized rooms with a standard weight limit bed, when she should have been put in one of the large rooms with the extra weight capacity bed. Therefore, due to her body habitus, and where she was roomed, we were set up for failure from the get-go.

I entered the room and greeted her, realizing right away that the current table was inadequate to support her. I buzzed my staff and inquired if we could move her. They told me no because all the rooms were full. I sat down, positioned her, and began the examination. As she re-positioned herself on the table, I noticed, too late, that the back of the table was rising and before I knew it, the table and the patient were *on top of me*!

I couldn't reach the call button. The patient began to panic and started yelling at me that I needed to do something. She informed me that I should be comforting her right now because she was very scared. *She* was scared? I was pretty scared myself. I completely agreed but did not have enough breath to even call out, much less to reassure her. I was pinned down beneath her *and* the table!

I calmly asked the patient to call out for help instead. She just kept yelling at me that she couldn't hear me. I finally got out enough audible words so that she did hear me and called for help. The "weight" of irony was definitely upon me that day. Fortunately, a staff member finally heard her.

My poor, unsuspecting staff member opened the door, eyes bugging and came in and saw our predicament. "Jesus Criminy" were the only words that came out of her mouth before she ran to get help. Then several more staff members arrived and were able to lift her and the table off me.

No one was harmed, thank goodness, including myself, but it was startling to say the least. Worse than that, it was unnecessary. If the office wasn't so jammed full, we could have switched rooms or placed her in a proper room in the first place. Situations like this contributed to my decision to go solo instead.

10

BUT, WHAT ABOUT MY HUSBAND?

One day, in my busy group practice, I was seeing OB patients. One of my postpartum patients was concerned about her breast milk, worried she was not producing enough. I performed an exam, which exhibited normal results. Both nipples were lactating as expected. There were no inversions or skin lesions.

I asked her all the usual questions:

- Could she hear the baby swallowing? *"Yes."*
- Did the baby still seem hungry after eating? *"No."*
- Was the baby still fussy after eating? *"No."*
- How often was she doing feedings? *"Every two to four hours."*
- Was she feeding from both sides? *"Yes, equally."*

She gave all the reassuring answers. I told her that it sounded like everything was going as it should. We weighed the baby, and the baby was gaining weight appropriately. She nodded, but still didn't seem reassured. I asked her if there was anything else she was worried about. She paused for a minute and then asked, "Well, what about my husband?"

It took me a minute, and then suddenly I flashed on an image of her husband on one breast and her baby on the other. I composed myself and asked, "What do you mean? What *about* your husband?". She looked at me with large doe eyes and said, "Well, sometimes he gets thirsty too." I realized my vision had been correct.

Ever the professional and avoiding a condescending tone - because she was serious - I said, with understanding and confidence, "I am sure that your husband has enough alternative fuel sources that he need not compete with your infant. Let's leave the milk for the baby and I am sure you will not have any more issues." She smiled broadly, thanked me, and left the office.

I found myself glad to help and more than a little concerned it was an issue in the first place...

PART III

PRIVATE PRACTICE

11

HOW DOES IT WORK?

After a year and a half off as a stay-at-home mom, I had exhausted my group practice opportunities. I'd unsuccessfully searched for work a reasonable distance from my home and interviewed with all the local practices, but I didn't get anywhere. I decided to strike out on my own. While I treasured all my time with my baby girl, there were bills that needed to be paid and education that was ready to be put to use. It was time to get back to work.

I had met with almost everybody in town and they all seemed interested, but we really couldn't get on the same page. I took that as a sign. It was time to start my own practice.

Now, here's the thing: I had no idea what I was doing. Another crucial education opportunity was missed during residency - we weren't trained for the business side of medicine. I think residency professors assume the majority of residents are going to move on to an established practice so it's really not a concern. Believe me, it's a concern! I had never started a practice before.

Now, I had to apply for all my licenses again, establish an address, redo all my accreditations, confirm credentials with insurances so I could get paid, pay bills, hire and fire staff, find an office manager, find a biller, and order equipment and software. This preceded the days of electronic medical records and all *those* requirements, and there was still that much to do! *Oh, my lord!* I had never done any of this on my own before.

And then, I got really lucky. I was still in touch with my old medical assistant from my group practice and she was looking for a new job. She also had a friend who was an office manager at another practice who knew all about running a practice. Before you know it, off we went. We started off from scratch, squeaked by on a tiny budget, relatively speaking, and just hung on until money started coming in, which wasn't for about three months.

You see, another thing we weren't taught is that you cannot just start a business to make money. You have to *have* money first to be able to even start the business. Then, you need enough money to survive until the business starts making money. It's trickier than you think.

Having said that, I am still so glad that I pivoted to private practice. Yes, every responsibility is mine now. Every paycheck, every bill, every outcome, everything. When something goes right, you get to rejoice. When something goes wrong, you are left holding the bag. There are no set hours. You are on call for you, 24 hours a day, seven days a week. The other side of that coin is that you can be assured of the quality of care you provide 100% of the time because you are the only one giving it. It's a trade off I was more than willing to accept, and still do.

I USED TO WEAR PIGTAILS

I had always been told that I looked young for my age. This was consistently frustrating when I was *actually* young, then got interesting, and then flattering as I got older. I started to wonder how much my appearance affected my patients' and their families' ability to take me seriously. I decided to test my theory. Ever the fan of a social experiment, I started wearing my hair in ponytails about 50% of the time when I operated.

This served two purposes: first, it provided a small but significant reduction in sweating to death in the operating room and second, it allowed me to conduct my experiment and see if there was a difference in patient and family reaction to what I had to say. Let me just say that my suspicion was validated. There was a definite difference.

I can remember one emergency surgery that I performed for a patient with an ectopic (tubal) pregnancy. The patient came in with a ruptured tube, bleeding significantly and required emergency surgery. Fortunately, the surgery was successful, and the patient did well. I went to speak to the family afterward, ponytails flapping in the breeze.

I tried to hedge my bets by wearing my doctor lab coat and having my medical badge clearly visible. I explained the surgery and outcome in detail. I went on to discuss post operation restrictions and what this meant for future pregnancy possibility. They all listened with rapt attention, which I thought was good.

I asked them if they had any more questions before I went back to check on the patient. The patient's mother then said, "That is all wonderful, dear, but when is the actual doctor coming to speak to us?" *The actual doctor?*

I smiled politely, pointed to my badge, and said, "Well, as it turns out, I *am* the actual doctor." There was a collective gasp and some murmured apologies. I assured them it was fine, that it happened all the time. I asked them to let me know if they needed anything else and gracefully excused myself. I decided no more pigtails. I would have to go back to sweating... *oh, well.*

13

"NO WORRIES, I'VE GOT THE MAP"

Over the last 20 years, I have had the privilege of treating many homosexuals, heterosexual, bisexual, pansexual, transexual, transgender, and gender fluid women. I have learned immensely from all of them and found each relationship fascinating in its own way. I have done my best to help them embrace their authentic selves and live their lives the healthiest way possible.

I noticed over the years that in my patient population, I cannot speak for others, some of my same sex partner patients have a slightly possessive relationship. I didn't realize how far this extended until I saw a certain couple one day – and got a good laugh out of it.

The patient was presenting some issues with pain with intercourse and some vaginal irritation. Her partner came with her and sat in the room during the exam. I positioned the patient, and she began telling me what her issue was. I started examining her while asking her questions when suddenly her partner jumped up and came over to me and started manipulating the patient's genitals, demonstrating to me where to look for the problem.

She informed me that she "had the map" and had "explored the area thoroughly many times" so she should be the one to show me what the problem was. The patient was embarrassed, to say the least. I then looked up and smiled sweetly at the patient's partner and said, "No worries. I happen to have the same map. I think I will be just fine. Thank you for your help." Fortunately, she sat down then and let me finish my job.

14

THE SINGING SURGEON

I have seen a lot of YouTube videos over the years where doctors sing to their patients, especially those delivering babies. Well, I am here to tell you I have been singing to patients *long* before it was "cool" or posted to any social platform.

I have sung Happy Birthday to every newborn baby and their parents for over 20 years. I have not missed a one. Sometimes it is all of us singing together: the OB staff, nurses, anesthesia, parents, and myself. Sometimes it is just me. Sometimes they video. Sometimes they don't.

I also take this a step further and I sing to some of my OR patients, too, just before they drift off to sleep. They say it helps them have nicer anesthesia dreams. Not everybody wants it, so I don't do it all the time, but I feel like it is a nice little gesture. Sometimes, it's the small details that can really make a difference in patient experience.

BUT YOU'RE SUCH A GOOD TEACHER, AND YOU DON'T STOMP AND SCREAM!

Here's the typical lead in: "Doc, we have a bunch of new staff today and some of them are still learning to use the robot. We thought we would put them all in your room since you are such a good teacher. We knew you wouldn't mind."

I used to love hearing those words. I mean, I still do. To me, it's validation I know my job so well that I can help others learn, which will in turn help me do my job better. Another interpretation is that I don't make a scene like an asshole when something does not go my way. (Believe me, I feel like my good behavior is become more the anomaly nowadays, which is disappointing.)

I always figure that if you are not willing to teach others, then you cannot expect people to follow your lead and you have no right to blame others when they don't. I love to teach. it is one of my favorite things. It is a big part of my job. Further, it can never be a bad thing that you don't behave like a jerk.

However, that phrase has become a bit of a double-edged sword in the past several years. Now, instead of it being a compliment, it has become more of a punishment. It has become indicative of an assumption by my OR staff that they can put any student or staff in my room - even if they do not know what they are doing. They know I will teach that team member and get through the operation, what we call a "case", somehow.

It doesn't matter if it doubles the time–to finish the case or causes frustration for me. They know I will not "have a cow" or make a scene over it. I am fine with teaching; I just don't want my reputation for patience and teaching to work against me. I would like to finish a case in a timely manner sometimes.

The phrase "the squeaky wheel gets the grease" seems to apply wherever I go and wherever I work. To me, it is illogical. Continuing to respond to those squeaky wheels only perpetuates bad behaviors; it doesn't remediate them. So, I say we put an end to it and reward us nice guys for a change.

Just sayin.'

16

THAT TIME I WAS SECRETLY IN LABOR

Let me take you back to 2004. I was "significantly" pregnant with my second daughter at 36 weeks (remember, full term is 40). I was working non-stop as a solo OBGYN. The pregnancy was going well once I had my gestational diabetes under control. It was business as usual. I was healthy and feeling good.

I was heading down to the operating room for what I thought was going to be a routine abdominal hysterectomy. At that point in time, early in my career, the average hysterectomy would take me about an hour or so at most. I suspected this patient would be no different, based on the available history I had at the time. The key word here is "available."

I scrubbed in with one of my colleagues and we got to work. Just as I was making my initial incision, I started getting a few "twinges" in the hinterland's region. Yes, they were in fact contractions. I figured they were just Braxton hicks. You know, the practice fakey contractions before the real ones happen. Even if they weren't, I figured I would have plenty of time to finish my surgery and deal with them later. It was only going to be an hour or so. This was only my second baby, and I was early - she was *not* ready to come yet... right?

I kept silent and kept going. I started to realize that I might be in trouble when I got through the fascia layers and into the peritoneum and saw that my patient's pelvis looked like a bomb had gone off inside. There were so many adhesions that you could barely see her organs! Adhesions are extensive connections between tissues that make organs and tissues stick together and significantly increase the complication of the surgery and increase the time it takes to dissect. As it turns out, the patient had neglected to inform me that she had had radiation with her colon cancer.

I would have benefitted from that reveal ahead of time so I could have planned better. Later, the patient said that she was sure it would not make a difference, so she left it out. *Oh sheesh.* This was *not* going to be just an hour. "Ok, no problem," I told myself, "just keep going."

As I was convincing myself there was no problem, my contractions started getting stronger and more frequent. I even started doing the mini-Lamaze breathing underneath my surgical mask. I am normally quite chatty during surgery and conversation quickly became impossible because I had to pause during contractions. Eventually, I just stopped talking all together and only motioned to my colleague and surgical tech when I needed something.

Did I speak up about what was going on? *Heck no!* I was determined to finish that surgery. I was not going to let my patient down!

Finally, three hours later, the surgery was done. Now I was really contracting, and I really couldn't hide it anymore. I quickly asked my colleague if he could write orders for me. He looked at me quizzically and asked, "Why?". I told him I needed to run upstairs for a second... (to have a baby, but he didn't need to know that). He agreed and I left, headed for labor and delivery.

I tried sneaking to my office first and putting myself on the monitor to see if I was really contracting or not. Apparently, I was not convinced. However, my office manager caught me before I got far and quickly realized that I was in labor. She sent me directly to labor and delivery.

Well, she was correct, and my daughter came by C-section later that day... and my colleagues and OR staff still never had any idea!

17

I HATE TO ADMIT IT, BUT SOMETIMES THERE IS SUCH A THING AS AN UGLY BABY

I t is said all babies are cute, no matter what. I went into the practice of OBGYN believing this statement with all my heart. I couldn't wait to be the first to lay hands on as many of those little preciouses as possible before ceremoniously handing up to their mothers. I was going to treasure all of their angelic faces in my memory forever.

Well, I am here to tell you that, in fact, all babies are not actually cute. Oh sure, the vast majority make you want to swoon right on the spot with their preciousness, perfect skin, and big blue eyes. And then, there are the others. There are the newborns who look like a wrinkled and plucked chicken. There are the newborns who look like a hairy little monkey. There are the newborns who have the most attractive parents you have ever seen, and you find yourself scratching your head at the combination of their features that greets you.

So, the question remains, what is the proper etiquette here? You deliver that one surprise wrinkled monkey baby and what do you say? Thank goodness for masks so if you slip up and change your facial expression, no one can see it.

You have to say something, though. My usual is, "Happy

Birthday! Welcome to the world, Gorgeous!" Now, when monkey baby comes out, I find myself saying something like, "Happy Birthday! Well look at you!" So, still nice, just maybe not including the "gorgeous" part.

I just want to remind everyone that this does not apply 100% of the time. Of course, I do not really have a script. I sometimes say, "Look at you!" with the cute babies, too. So, for those of you who may have heard this from me over the years, it is not some automatic code for ugliness - please don't worry. Even if they were ugly at the beginning, they all get cuter with time.

Ya just gotta age them a little bit.

18

THE OLD LADIES AND THE UNDERWEAR

One day I had one of my geriatric patients ask me, "Doctor, can I show you something?" Of course, I said yes, and she proceeded to remove her underwear to show me some crusty yellow substance that had collected in it. She said, "This has been going on for a while. I thought I should ask you what it is?" Yup. That's my job. I know, I know. But... *ewww?*

Even this scenario has a teachable moment. Do not say an immediate "Yes" when a patient asks to show you something! Ask for some clarification to prepare yourself first. I have been shown everything from crusty underwear and necrotic lesions to fungus toenails. I get it, that is the nature of my business and I do embrace that wholeheartedly. I am just saying that sometimes I need a minute to "get ready." I have learned the hard way to pause before giving a knee jerk "yes" or "no" to every question I have been asked in the last 25 years.

Here's another important example: when someone says "Doc, can I leave my socks on because I just came from the gym?" I want to say "no" because I like to examine their feet as part of the checkup. However, the correct answer should be "yes" out of self-preservation because they are trying to give me a heads up that I am not prepared for the extreme FO (foot odor) that I am about to experience because their feet *will* be in my face.

PART IV

LESSONS LEARNED ALONG THE WAY

19

RECOMMENDATIONS, SCHMECKOMMENDATIONS

There is nothing that frustrates me more than confusing guidelines for women. Let's take for example the current PAP smear guidelines. Current pap smear guidelines suggest that women can space out their pap smears every couple of years after the age of 30 Further, these guidelines suggest women don't need a PAP smear until the age of 21.

These recommendations make sense from a purely epidemiologic, statistical standpoint. However, in my opinion, they are terrible from a practical standpoint. Here is why: Nearly every time I try to follow these guidelines, someone gets hurt.

For example, I had a perfectly healthy 30-year-old patient with no significant history, safe sexual practices and no history of abnormal paps. Per national guidelines, she hadn't had a pap in three years... and she also hadn't had an exam in that same time because she thought no pap meant no checkup. Technically, she was not incorrect.

Well, when she showed up three years later, she had invasive cervical carcinoma. She needed a radical hysterectomy and radiation. It changed her life forever. It ended her ability to have more children. She had to put her new job on hold. Fortunately, she persevered and survived and is very successful today.

The thing is, when I was doing her exam that day, I knew she had cancer the moment I looked at her cervix. I also knew that it didn't pop up overnight. My heart sank as I realized that this was preventable and could have been caught much earlier when the solution would have been much simpler.

This is what I am talking about - people get hurt with these recommendations. I don't care if it is only a handful who are outliers. I don't care if it is more cost effective to practice medicine this way. What is more costly than an unnecessary loss of life? I can't think of anything. They are still people, and they count.

These guidelines for women are confusing, unclear, and incomplete. The recommendations only refer to the actual pap smear, but they get interpreted to encompass all gyn care. Because of the lack of clarity, women interpret these recommendations to mean that they don't even need an annual gyn checkup anymore.

This is potentially harmful for multiple reasons. First, the pap smear is only about 20 seconds of what goes on at an annual visit. The rest of the visit entails a head-to-toe exam and discussion of multiple health issues. Second, when women miss the opportunity for this essential checkup, they miss the opportunity to notice gyn issues while they are still small issues instead of life-threatening problems.

The wonderful thing about most OBGYN medical issues is that they can often be picked up with just routine surveillance. The scary thing is most OBGYN medical issues do not exhibit symptoms until things are advanced and life-threatening. Ovarian cancer can just present with a little constipation and decreased appetite. Uterine cancer can present with a little bleeding in between periods or after menopause.

Without a headlamp and significant contortionist abilities, there is no way to be able to fully self-assess for gyn issues until it may be too late. It's just not possible! There is nothing more heartbreaking than giving bad news to someone that is at risk of dying from a totally preventable condition.

Bottom line: please just give me 20-30 minutes of your time once a year and I will do my darndest to make sure you are ok. I care about your future! Give me a chance to make sure you have one.

20

REINVENTING MYSELF

When you come out of medical school and residency, you are positively ebullient that the hard stuff is over, and life is ready to begin again. You are ready to start your practice, whether that be with a group, an employed position, or going solo. You can't wait to practice medicine and help as many people as you can and make a difference in the world. That first set of patients can't arrive soon enough!

As you know, I opted – eventually - for solo practice. I tried group employment first and it didn't work out, so I set up my own practice. I knew it was the right move for me.

Wow! What I didn't know, was that none of my training had prepared me to handle the business of medicine, the hassle of insurances, or the ins and outs of running a practice by myself. I didn't realize the rest of my career would not just be about the blissful, soul-fulfilling practice of medicine using my best medical judgement to achieve the best outcomes. It would be a struggle for balance between practicing medicine, battling with insurances, paying bills, hiring, firing, and not taking your work home with you.

Having said that, as a solo, your work is always with you. You are on call 24/7 and your main back up is you. I knew that going in but that doesn't mean it's not tough sometimes. Still, for me, it is a worthy trade off for knowing that I can be 100% assured of the quality of care for my patients.

I thought going into medicine I would practice the same way for my whole career, focusing on the same types of issues and methods. I was *so* wrong. The practice of medicine is constantly evolving, and you must evolve with it.

I am constantly studying and learning and offering new options and services. I go to conferences to learn the latest and greatest OBGYN updates. Actually, with the pandemic, conferences have become scarce, so I'm on more webinars and zooms lately.

I can't believe how many new medications come out every year. The number of new surgical techniques I have learned over the years is astonishing. Now that I am an accomplished robotic surgeon, I do everything minimally invasive and I even send home hysterectomy patients home the same day, right from the recovery room! Back in the beginning, I did most hysterectomies abdominally.

To stay relevant, increase my bottom line, take away some of the control of insurances and provide more well-rounded services, I developed an aesthetic business as a complement to my OBGYN practice. As the world has started viewing patients more as clients, it has become even more imperative to offer extras, latest and greatest, and additional services to stay competitive - stay in business.

I learned that these service expansions were necessary to simply afford to practice what I originally studied in the first place. Now, I don't just offer OBGYN services. I offer laser hair removal, CoolSculpting, photo facials, Aviva scarless labiaplasty, Morpheus, micro needling, scar revision, stretch mark treatment, fat reduction, skin tightening, vaginal rejuvenation and I am adding more all the time.

Fortunately, I have been able to adapt. Otherwise, I could not stay in business. I take just as much pride in those additional offerings as I do with my general OBGYN practice.

21

THE SACRED RESPONSIBILITY OF SURGERY

Have you ever heard of the surgical pause before a procedure starts? The surgical pause occurs when everyone in the operating room stops what they are doing and pays attention to the circulator. The circulator then reads to the entire room the patient's name, date of birth, what surgery they are having, what antibiotics are being administered, any allergies the patient has, if the instruments have been properly sterilized, and any other pertinent patient info. This is the moment for everyone to regroup and reconfirm the plan for the surgery.

I like to add another level to this. I like to use this moment, not only to confirm the surgical plan, but to remind everyone in the room of the sacred responsibility that we are about to undertake. I think of it as a moment of reflection. I like to make sure everyone realizes the awesome amount of trust that patient has in all of us to allow us to put them under anesthesia and remove things from their body.

It's mind blowing when you think about it. There really isn't another scenario in which someone relinquishes so much control to another person. It needs to be respected. I just like to make sure that everyone in the room is thankful for the opportunity that patient has given us.

22

THE BEST COMPLIMENT I EVER RECEIVED

Several years into my private practice, I got a compliment from a patient that kind of blew me away. I had no idea what it meant at first. Thank God, the patient explained it to me -otherwise, I still might not get it.

She said, "You know, Doc, I love coming here. It's just like coming to my girlfriend's house." In my head, my brain just started spinning. "What?! Your girlfriend's house?! What the heck do you do at your girlfriend's house?" Thank goodness I didn't actually say any of those words.

The patient must have recognized the incredulous look on my face. She laughed and said, "No, Doc. Let me explain. I mean that you make me so comfortable, I feel like I can talk to you about anything."

Ok, that right there is the best thing I have ever heard to this day. It was the best compliment ever. I felt like I finally arrived. It has always been my goal to provide the best, most compassionate, complete care that I can. The way I do that is allowing my patients to open up about whatever they want.

When she said that, I knew that I was on the right track. I try to stay mindful of that comment every day to keep that comfort level going. I want my patients to always feel like they can tell me anything. Even if I don't understand it at first.

23

I AM WISER AND HAPPIER NOW THAN I HAVE EVER BEEN

I have learned so much over the years of my career. I have grown, aged, changed, adapted, and learned. I have worked through my diagnosis and treatment for lymphoma last year. I have worked through the pandemic. I have looked at my profession with a dynamic vision that pushes me every day.

I wrote this book to share with you and give you a glimpse into the last 20 years or so. I wanted to share the reality, the practicality, the growth, the evolution, the humorous and the poignant moments. I want you to really see what the life of a doctor can be like. We are human beings. We have ups and downs. We get tired. We deal with a lot. The struggle for balance is real. I strive to blend my roles as doctor, wife, mother, musician, and writer every day. Sometimes I succeed. Sometimes I don't.

Society associates being a doctor with being steadfast and strong, but this concept negates the necessity of change in the field of medicine. Medicine is constantly evolving, and doctors must be willing to change with it. This change requires thoughtfulness, intent, and the resources to facilitate it.

When I see the world through my physician eyes, I see people to help all around me. I see my duty as a voice of guidance and reason. I see the possibility of improving lives. I see the ability to educate and nurture. This book is part of that education.

ALSO BY DR. LAURA

OK, It's My Turn Now: A Doctor's Journey Through Cancer

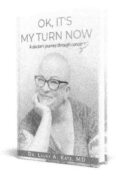

Dr. Katz has been a solo ob-gyn physician in Monroe, Michigan, for over twenty years. As if 2020 hadn't been challenging enough, she was saddled with a diagnosis of Hodgkin's Lymphoma in the midst of the COVID-19 pandemic. Undeterred, she decided to turn the tables on cancer. Armed with her usual overflowing positive attitude, she made it her mission to transform her experience into a metaphorical flashlight to guide other patients through cancer treatment. Using wit, grit, humor, and unabashed vulnerability, she gives us an intimate look into her personal journey.

ABOUT THE AUTHOR

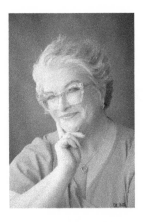

Dr. Laura Katz is a solo OBGYN in Monroe, MI where she lives with her husband and two daughters. She has been practicing medicine for over 20 years and has cared for women and girls of all ages with a wide range of health issues ranging from general OB care to cancer. She also owns a thriving aesthetic medicine business. She has made it her mission to care for and empower every woman she meets to live healthy and fulfilled, which is the same goal she sets for herself. When she is not practicing medicine, she actively volunteers with her local cancer support group, soaks up as much family time as possible, blogs, writes poetry, podcasts, and enjoys her garden.

RESOURCES

Find Dr. Katz around the web and on social media:

www.facebook.com/laurakdoc

Instagram.com/monroecomprehensivelasercenter This is the Instagram for the office and our aesthetic center. It has a little bit of everything.

Laurakdoc.blog This blog series is entitled Nothing's Off-Limits. We talk about a little bit of everything, except for politics!

Laurakatzmdpc.com This is the main office web page. It goes over everything that we do.

Straight Talk with Dr. Laura podcast can be found on Podbean and i Heart Radio. This is basically the audio version of the blog.

Facebook.com/groups/246607280530391 This is the Facebook group I created called Chemo Peeps. It is a peer group for anyone ever affected by cancer or cancer treatment in which patients, family, and friends can have real one-on-one discussions about everything cancer and share tips and stories.

CPSIA information can be obtained
at www.ICGtesting.com
Printed in the USA
BVHW030719200422
634790BV00005B/93

9 781950 476398